Sam Sloan Teaches A+

50 Helpful Questions

ISHI PRESS
INTERNATIONAL

Sam Sloan Teaches A+

50 Helpful Questions

First Edition

ISBN 0-923891-06-4
978-0-923891-06-0

Ishi Press International
1664 Davidson Avenue, Suite 1B
Bronx NY 10453
USA

917-507-7226

Printed in the United States of America

A+ 2007
50 Helpful Questions

by Sam Sloan

1.

You have installed a new hardware device and found the appropriate driver by the following steps

a. preforming a Google search and finding the correct driver
b. going to the manufacturers website and downloading the driver
c. digging through all of your cd collection looking for the cd that came with the device
d. going to a file sharing website such as Napster and performing a search of the driver

Answer: C Going directly to the manufacturers website is the only accepted approach. Drivers found on Google would only be downloaded from a third party source. Digging through all of you cd's is the approach of a very organized home user, but when working for a large office, employees are expected to download drivers directly from the manufacturers website of the hardware device. The last choice Napster is only helpful for downloading mp3's or maybe a nice movie, but not drivers.

2.

You are installing a driver for your new hardware device and receive the following message

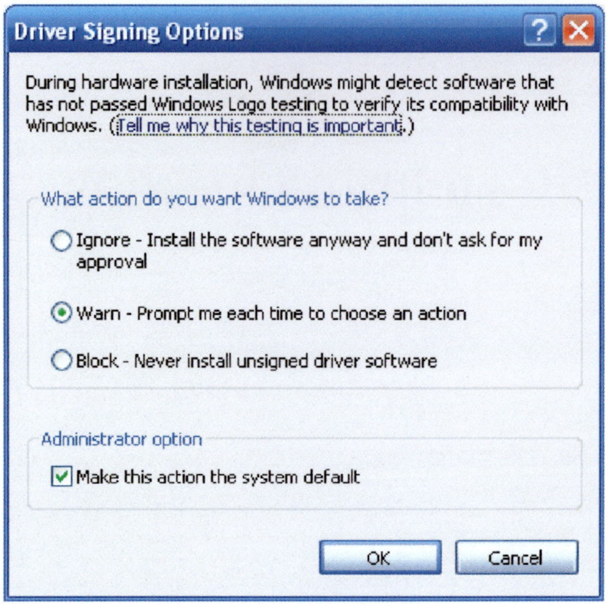

The question is asking which is the appropriate setting for allowing unsigned drivers

a. Ignore
b. Warn
c. Block

Answer: Block is the only acceptable answer for the entire exam. Any driver not signed directly by Microsoft Corp Although while working in the professional field you may encounter many drivers from trusted sources of downloads, when certifying with the A+ you are accepting the terms of your exam vendor. The official exam answer is only Microsoft signed drivers are accepted, all other drivers are blocked.

3.

You have installed a new driver for your modem and a error message appeared on your screen. After restarting your computer your modem no longer works. What steps need to be taken to resolve the problem

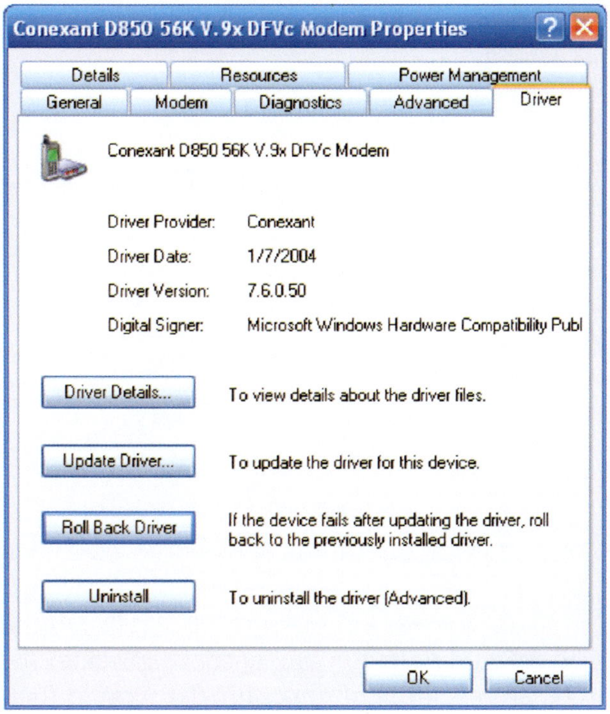

Answer: Roll back the driver. The update of the modem driver only updated one driver on the entire computer. There is a similar question which asks how to roll back all of the drivers on a computer after several months of updates. In this case we find the exact driver for this hardware device and Roll Back the exactly right driver. The question specified the driver for the modem, so we are only rolling back one driver, the modem driver.

4.

How do I find the device manager in Windows XP professional

There are two answers to this question,
Click< Start< Control Panel< System< Hardware

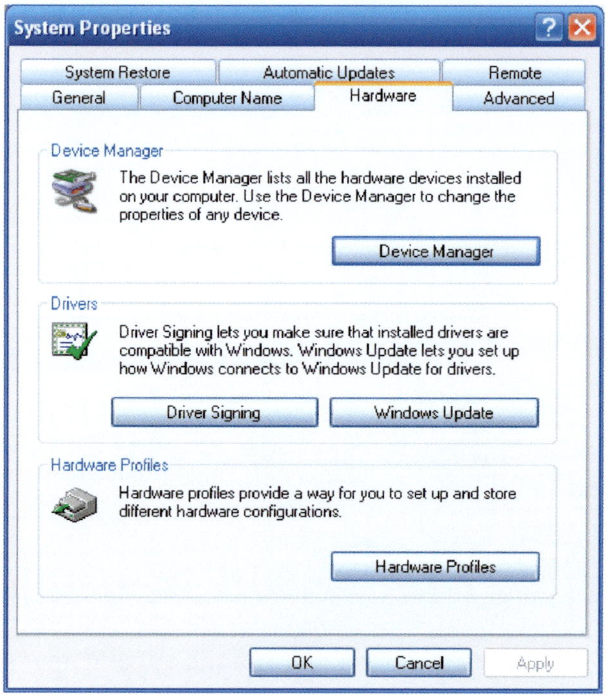

Click< Start

Right Mouse Click on My Computer and Select Manage

Select Device manager from the options on the left hand side.

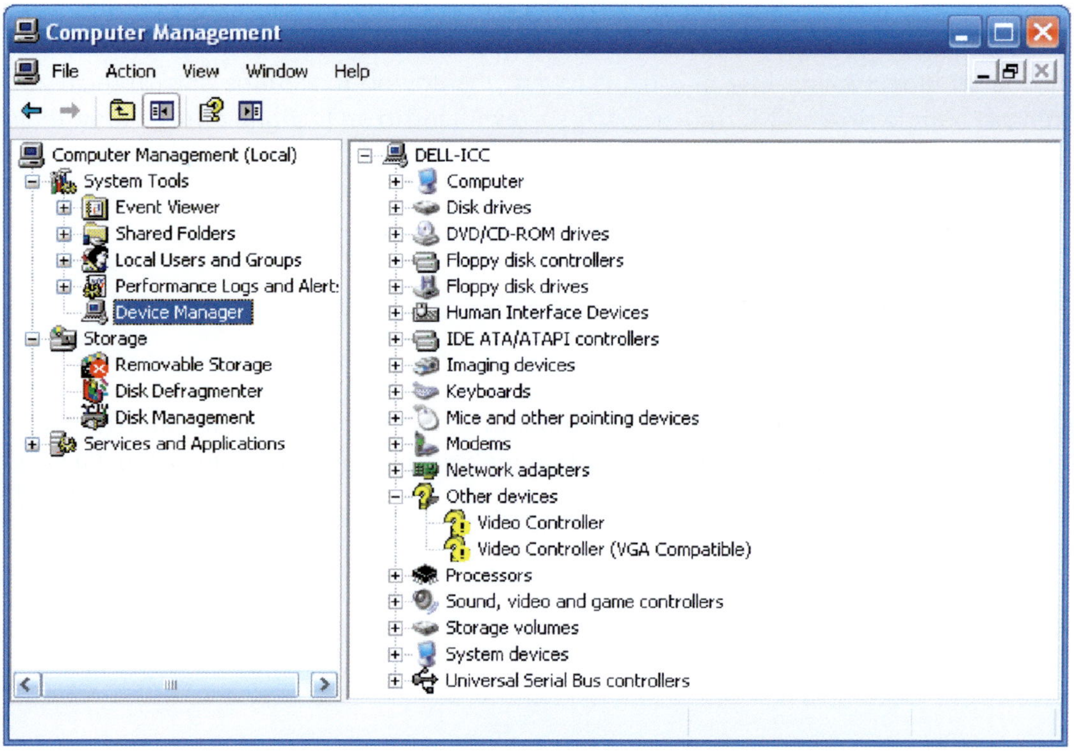

Remember the answer to this question is only to specify the path needed to find the device manager. No other information was asked for.

5.

There are several wordings of this question all asking for the name of the Computer Management Console

One wording asks for the name of the console that manages both Local Users and Computers and the Disk Defragmenter. Another wording asks for where to find the Device Manager using Computer Management Console. Another question asks how to reach System Tools using Computer Management Console, shown in the diagram below.

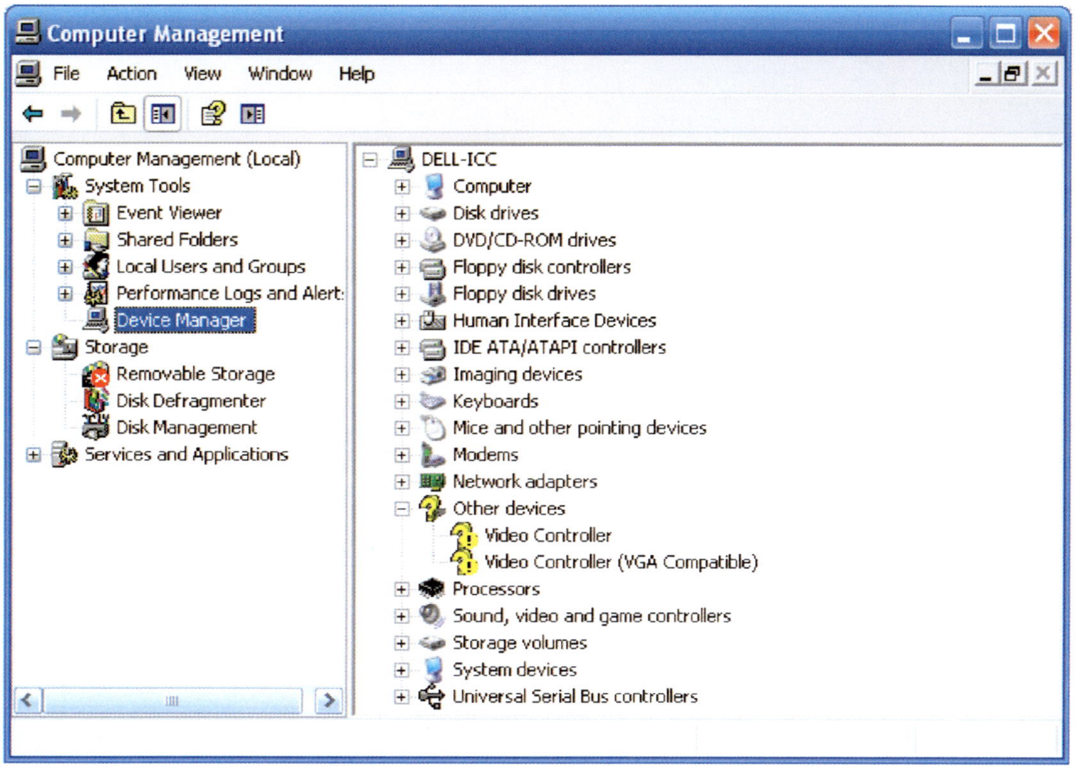

6.

You are about to install several new drivers and want to have assurance you can recover the computer if the computer starts to malfunction. What steps do you take

a. Run Backup Wizard and save all of the data on an external hard drive
b. Create a restore point for todays date
c. Burn all of the current settings on a DVD and the install the new drivers
d. Back up your registry settings from the command prompt

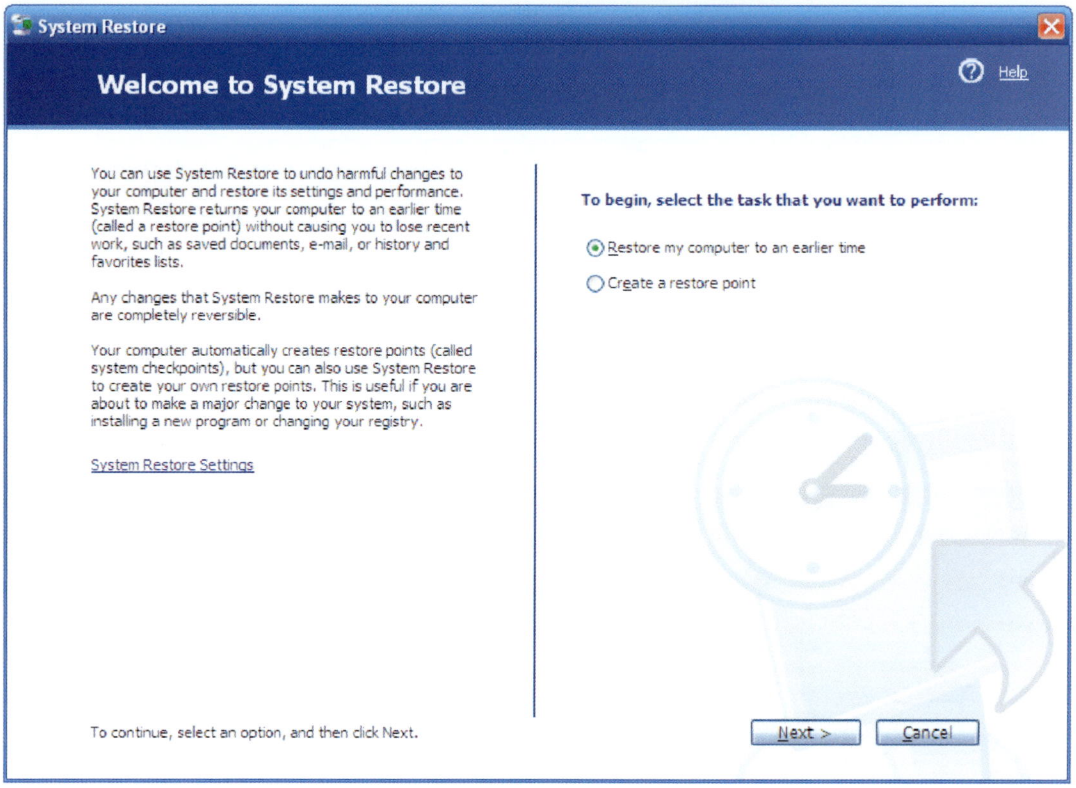

b. Creating a restore point will archive all of the drivers programs and documents included on your system. System Restore is found in the Help ans Support Icon from the Start menu. Backup wizard backs up data, not the current state of drivers. Burning all of your current setting on DVD is a trick question because there is only on DVD question on any A+ exam and the answer is 4 gigabytes. Backing up the registry is not a single question on the A+ exam. Registry settings are all backed up by todays software such as Norton. As of the year 2007 when this exam was written the help of IT is no longer needed to specialize in changing system registry's.

7.

Hardware profiles. There is one question specifically asking how a user can have a different driver configuration for using his laptop while traveling or using his laptop while at the office. Creating a hardware profile is the answer. Hardware profiles are located

Start< Control Panel< System< Hardware< Hardware Profiles

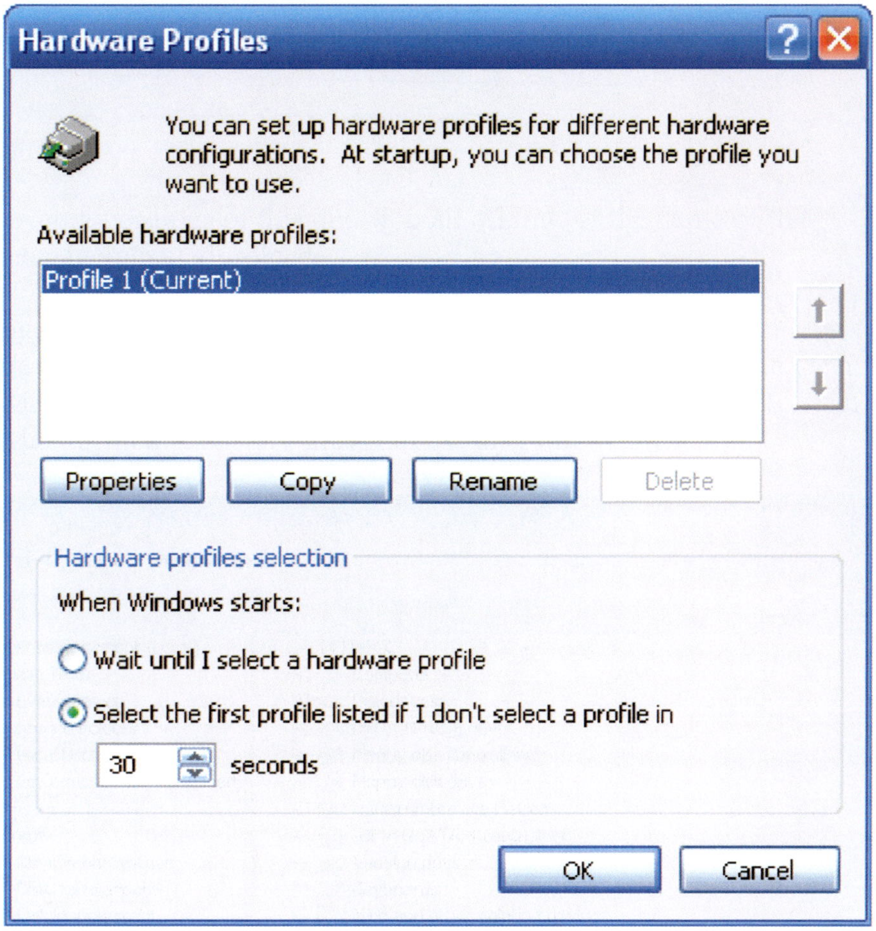

There is one similar question asking how to have a hardware profile start automatically when the computer is booted. The question makes it as if you are configuring for you boss at the office and do not want to inconvenience him by offering the wrong hardware profile. After all he writes your paycheck and wants his laptop working on his business trip. The answer is Select the profile in list

Set the time to 0 seconds.

A third hardware profile question asks about docked computers that need different profiles. Docked computers are always laptops. One definition of a docked station is a laptop that needs to connect to a different printer while at work then while at home.

<Start <Control Panel< System< Hardware< Hardware Profiles< Properties

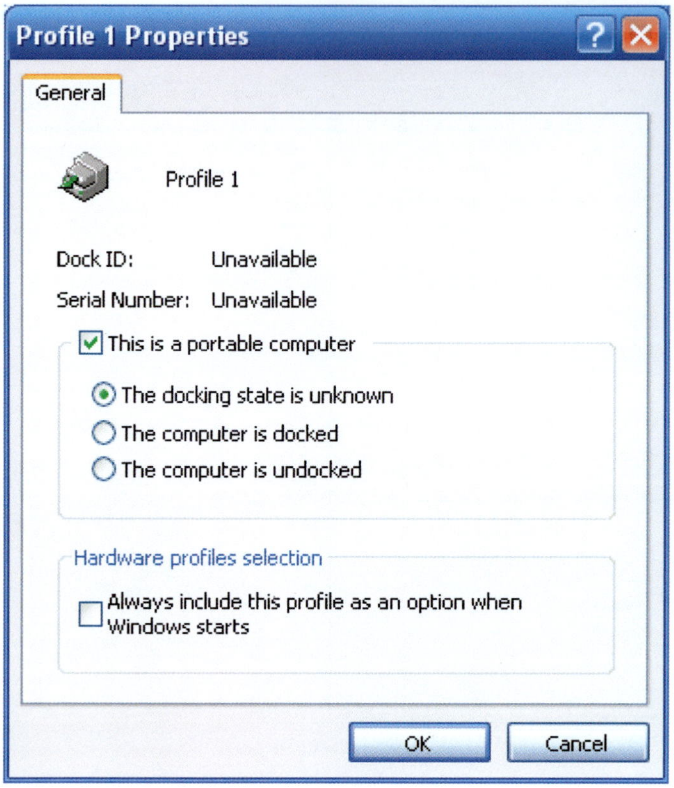

8.

Windows Update. This is not the same setting as automatic updates. Windows Update is located in System Properties< Under the hardware tab< In the drivers section < by clicking Windows Update

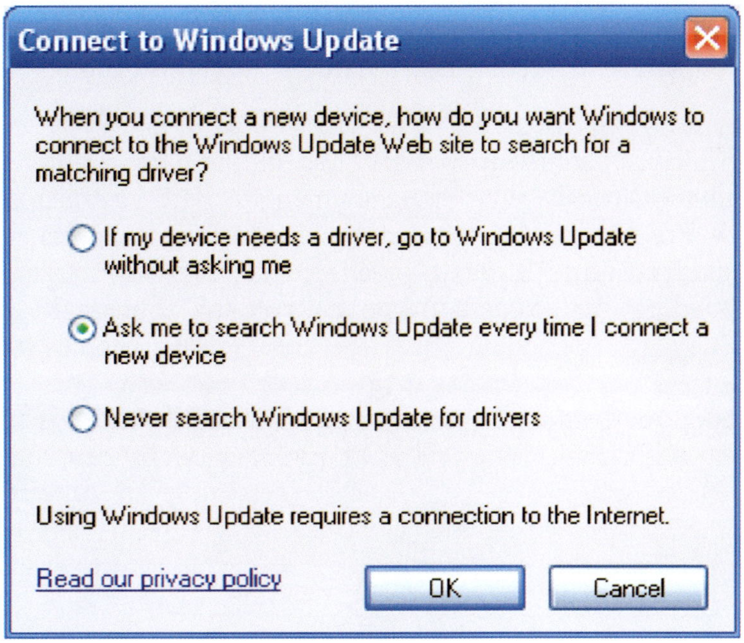

If you see this question anywhere during your exam, the answer is to go to Windows Update without asking me. While this approach is not recommended at the office, and as an IT administrator you should only allow changes to your company machines when needed, our A+ exam is catering to a vendor that requires all updates from Microsoft are trusted.

9.

We covered drivers that need to be rolled backed one at a time, or drivers that need to be archived with a Restore Point. There is one other sequence of drivers not working not discussed.

The question will ask how to return drivers to there previous state after a complete system crash. This is called the Last know good configuration. This is used when the system starts up and you need to restore your computer to the last set of drivers that worked for your machine. Last known good is brought about by restarting your computer and clicking f2 while your computer is running its Power On Self Test. Press the f2 button before the Windows startup screen appears.

Last Know good Configuration question always describes a complete system crash after installing a new driver.

10.

When your computer starts up a login screen appears showing several different user names to click on, each requiring a password. You would like to enable only one user account to be used at any time to save memory being used by too many programs running at once.

Click< Start< Control Panel< User Accounts< Change the way users log on or off

This is known as fast user switching.

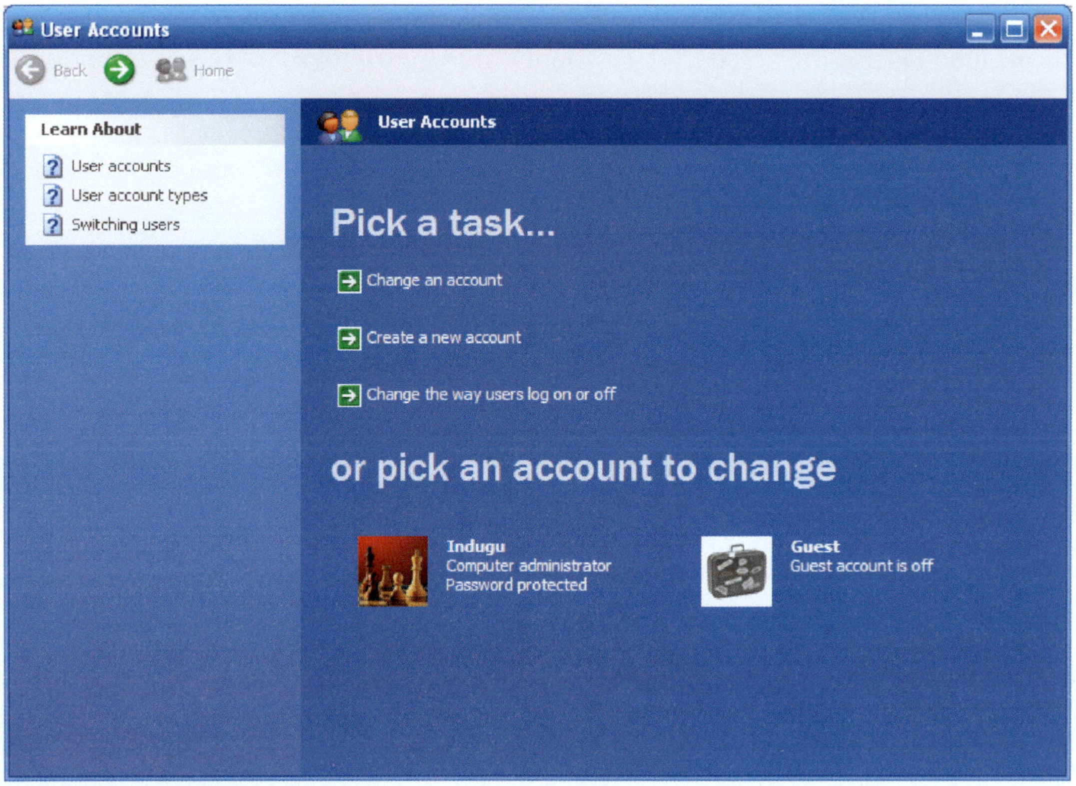

This will bring you to a screen with two check boxes. Uncheck the box for Use Fast User Switching. Click Apply Options

11.

There is a second and very similar question asking how to require the user name be typed in when logging in

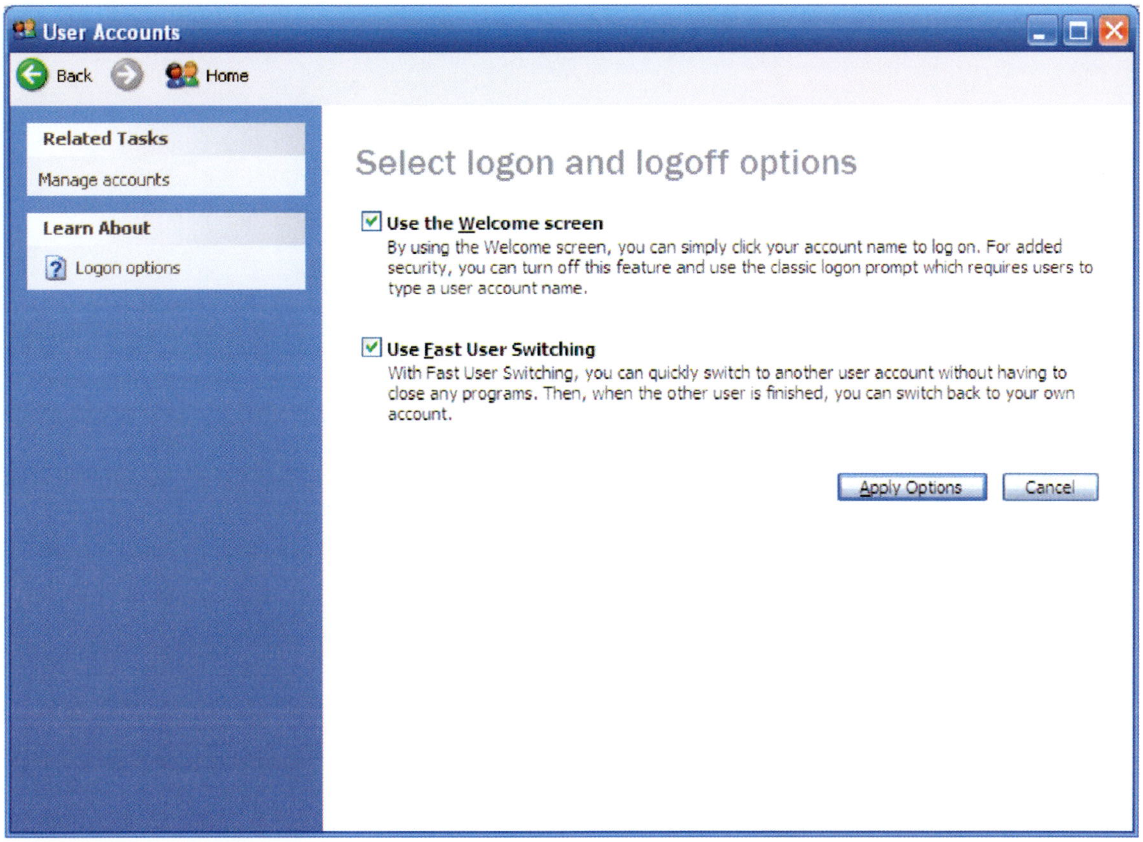

Click< Start< Control Panel< User Accounts< Change the way users log on or off< two check boxes are available. UnCheck< Use the Welcome Screen. This will make account names not visible to other users at your computer.

12.

Use Fast User Switching is a second question asking how to enable a computer for access to offline files and folders. Fast user switching must be turned off for offline files to be enabled. This requires one restart.

13.

TCP/ IP cards. The common question gives an example of the computer Internet connection not able to start. The question may ask for what device needs an updates driver, in which case you will be updating the Network Interface Card. NIC card drivers are found on the manufacturer website.

14.

Another question about NIC cards will be phrased asking how to start an new Internet connection for the first time.

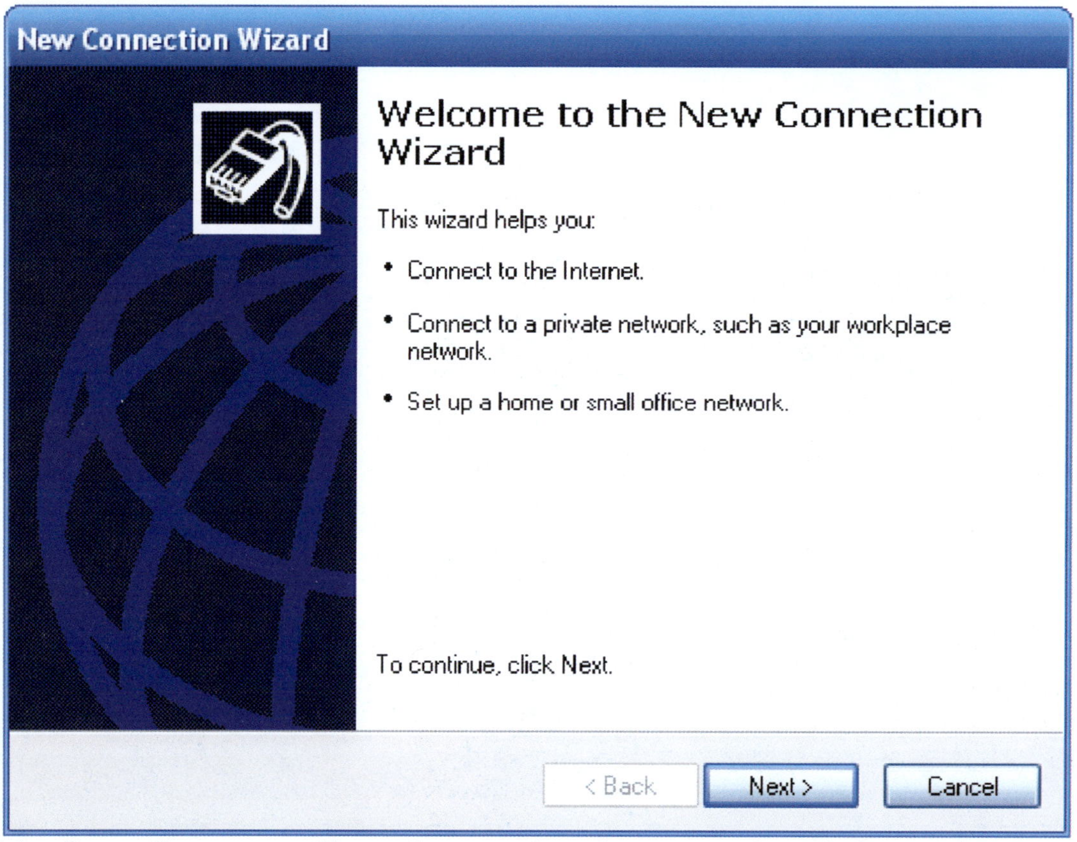

Click< Start< Connect to< Show all connections (or commonly called network connections)
Click< Create a New Connection

The A+ exam focuses very much on which button to click first. So this is already your complete answer. The remainder of the screens clicking through are not part of the answer. That is for the Network+ exam.

15.

Using the same New Connection Wizard another task asks how to setup a broadband connection also known as TCP/ IP.

Click< Start< Connect to< Show All Connections< Create a New Connection< Click Next< Select< Setup connection manually

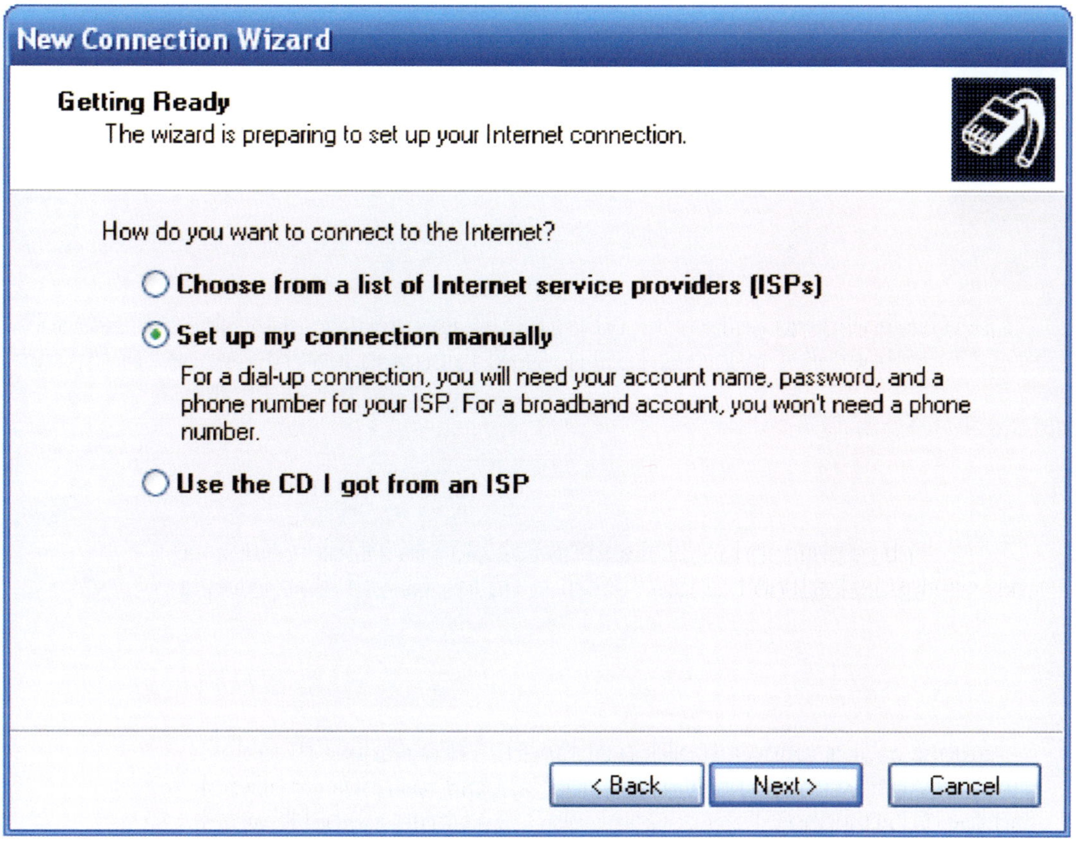

The next screen will be asking whether or not to use modem, DSL with a password or a broadband connection that is always on. We will choose the third option.

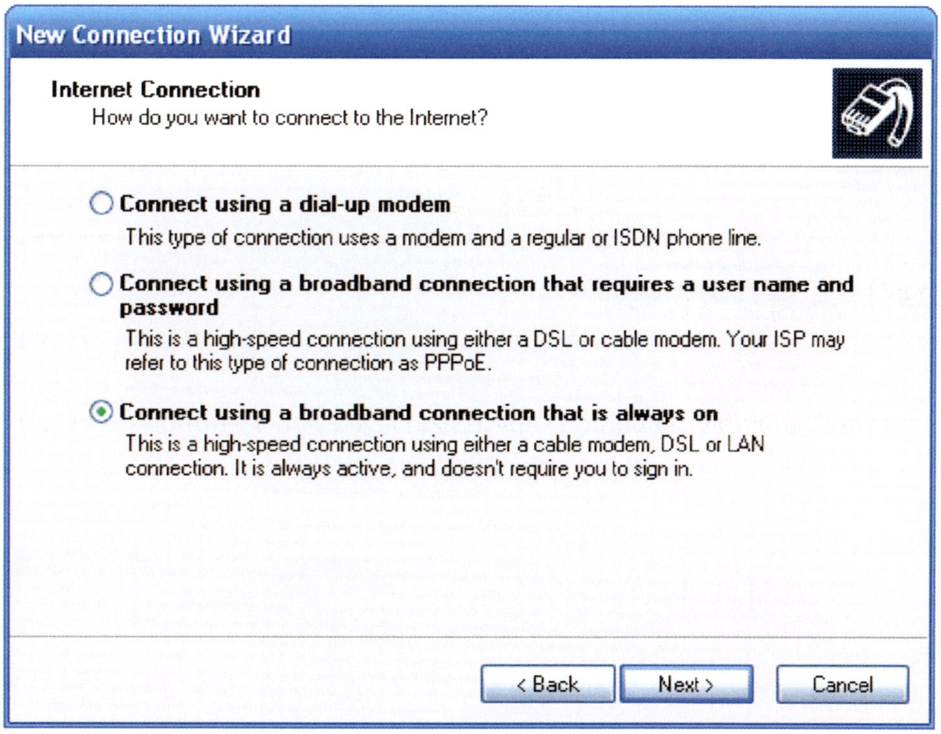

Click< Next< Click Finish Your Broadband Internet is now enabled.

16.

There is a short question on installing VPN connections. Remember the A+ is very much on the surface. The answer to installing VPN is clicking Start< Connect to< Show All Connections< Create a new Connection< Click Next< Click the second option Connect at my Office< Select the second option virtual Private Network connection.

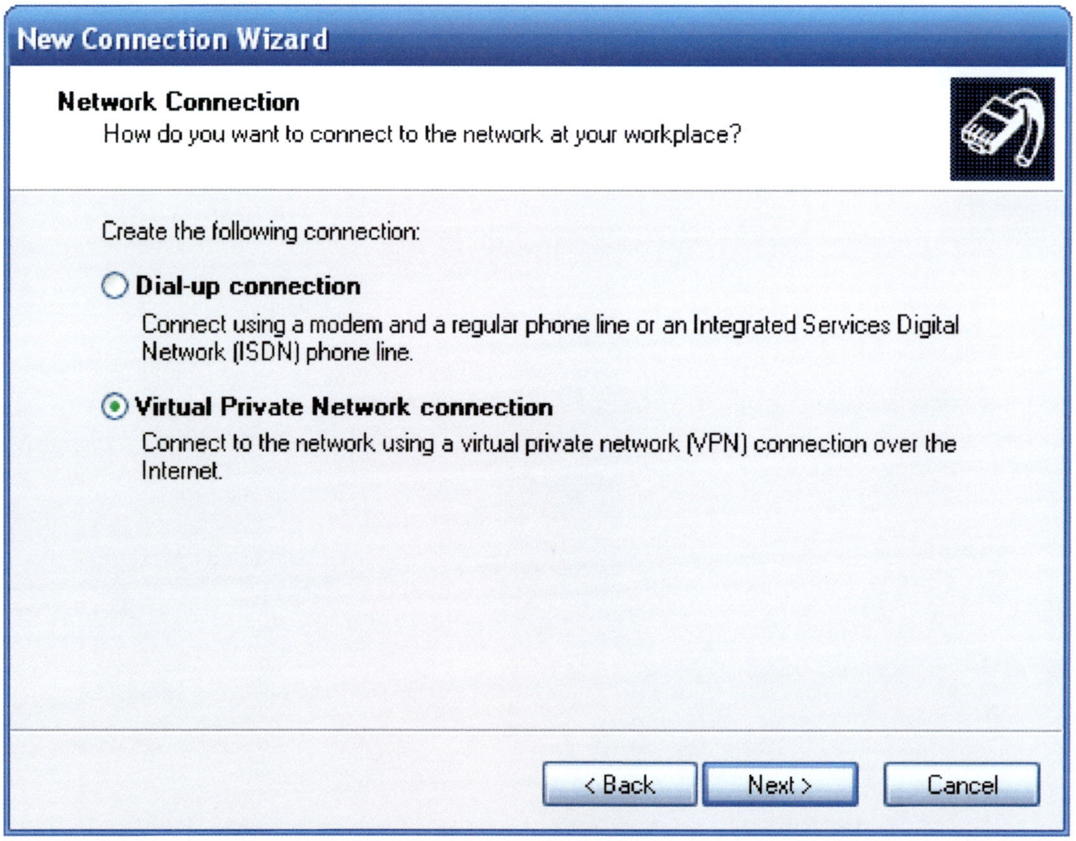

On the next screen select not to dial the initial Internet connection< Then type in the IP address of your company network. IP addresses are found by asking at your office help desk. They are remote connections and require that your office have a server that has tremendous bandwidth to enable remote users.

17.

A+ requires identifying computer parts here we will identify an IP address apart from a Mac

address and a

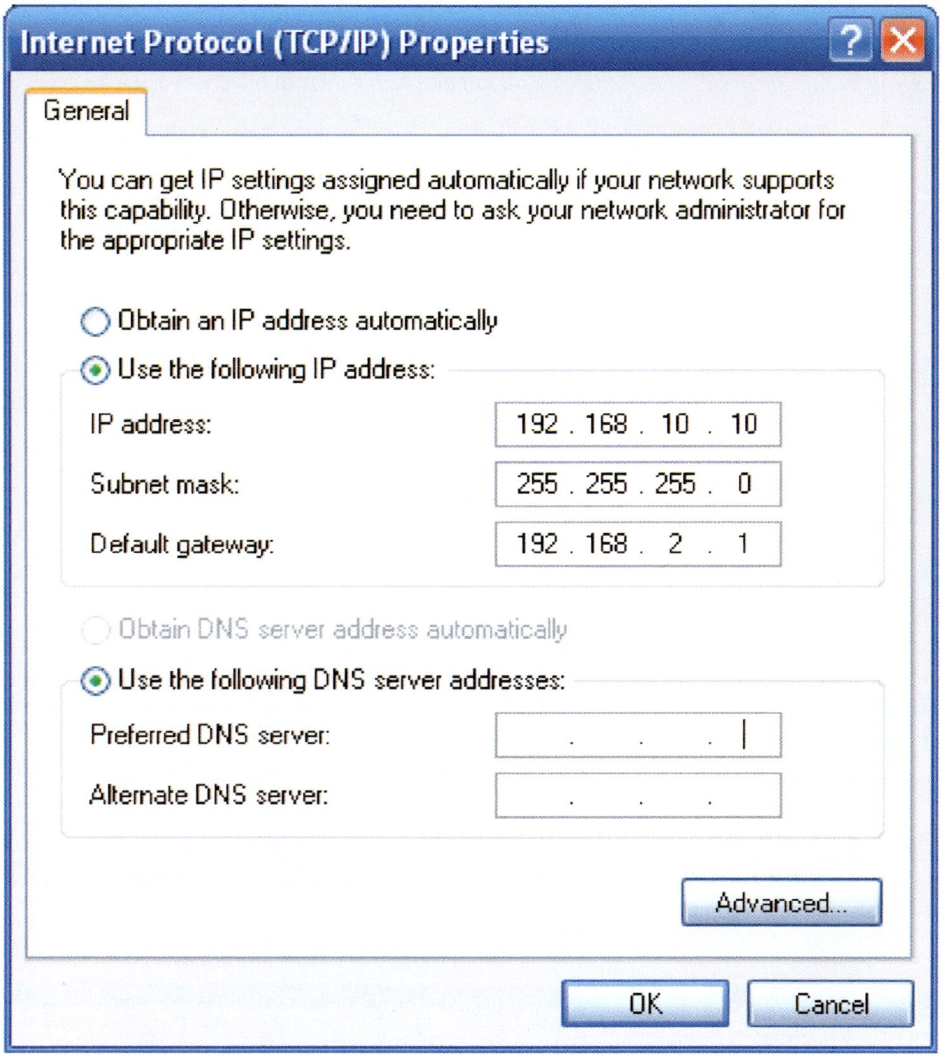

Click< Start< Connect to< Show All Connections< Local Area Connection< right mouse click <Properties< General tab< Scroll Down to TCP/ IP< Click properties<

In answer to this question the IP configuration is located in the properties of your network connection. Now three question will follow.

18.

By default a Broadband Internet connection will obtain an IP address automatically. You should leave this setting unchanged unless you are logging your computers Internet connection into an office network.

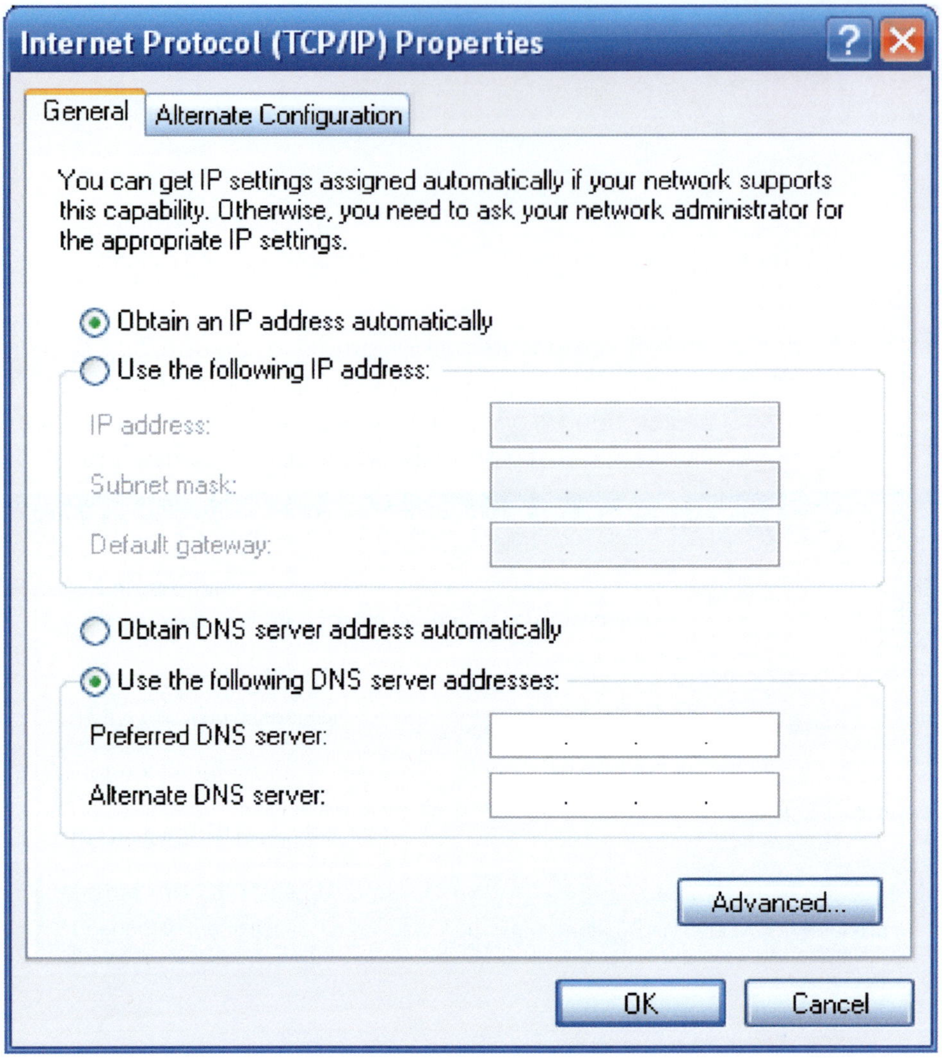

19.

Identify an IP address from a Subnet Mask. This is a very simple question. You will be asked 192.168.1.1

a. IP address
b. Subnet Mask

The answer is easy enough to remember. All of the Subnet mask's on the exam start with 255.255.255.0 for a class C subnet mask. So that leaves us with only one answer, this is an IP address. This is extremely important to identify because you may have to use them every day at the office. At my current job all of the printers are identified by and IP so users can print remotely.

20.

Identify class A B and C subnet masks.
Class A is 255.0.0.0
Class B is 255.255.0.0
Class C is 255.255.255.0
Class D is not on the exam.

21.

Identify a loopback address.
A loopback adapter tests if an NIC card is working or not. The answers 172.0.0.0 is the IP that will show up when pinging a loopback adapter.

22.

Identify what IP address decides when a Network Card is not working
169.254.0.0
That is the entire answer. When pinging a machine this error code means either the server DHCP network is down or the PC's network card is down. This is a very bad sign and you would not be able to proceed with installation.

23.

Identify the IP address of the gateway
192.168.1.1
The IP ends with 1.1, the gateway address on this exam always ends with 1.1 whether it be
185.231.1.1
185.231.1.10 (wrong)
185.231.1.9 (wrong)
A gateway is commonly a router that is attached to the computer.

24.

How do I install a Network printer.

Click< Start< Printers and Faxes< Printer Tasks< Add a Printer

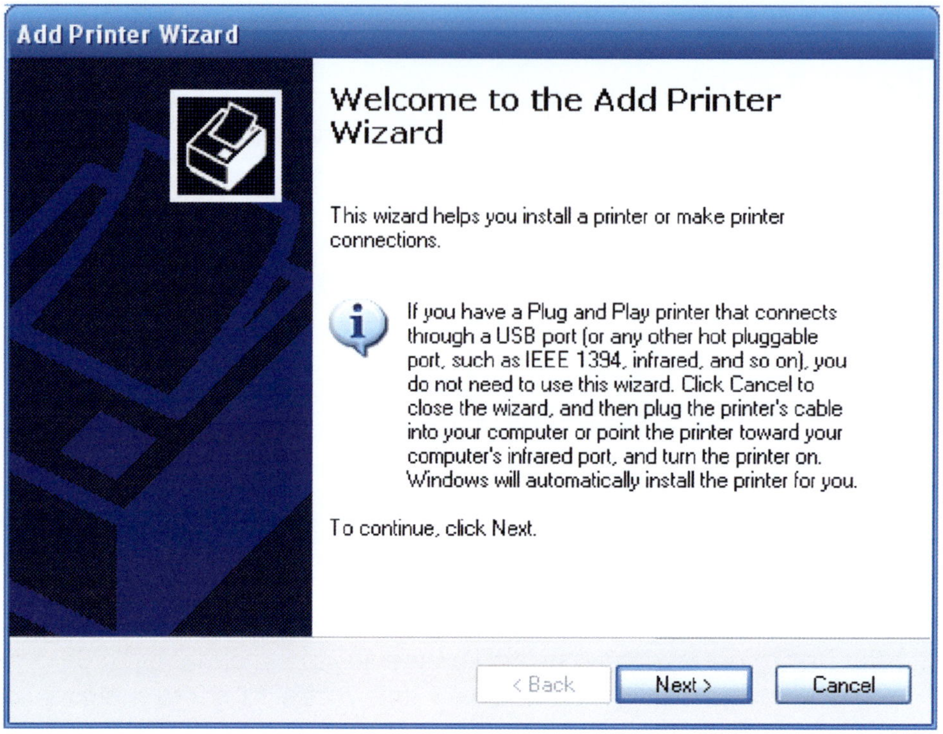

Click< Add a Network Printer

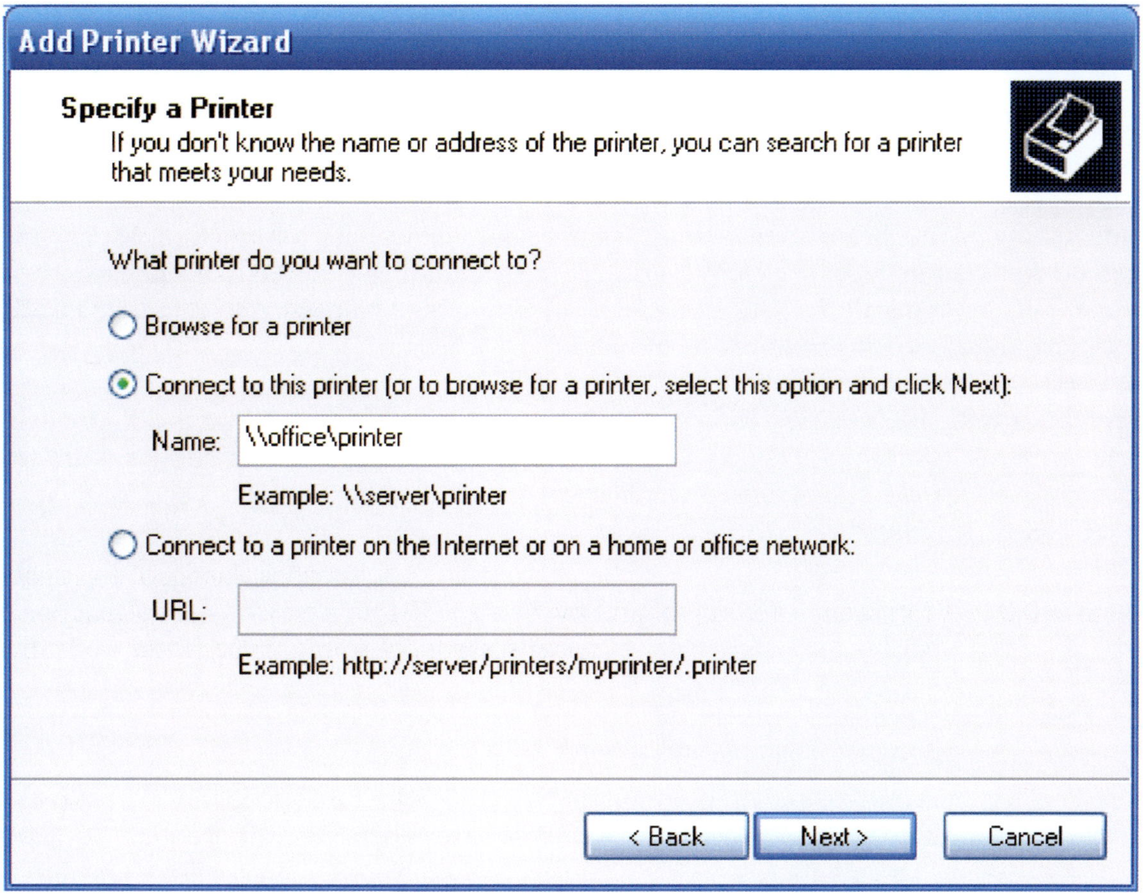

In the display shown either type in the IP address or the server URL of the printer. If the IP address does not match then you will get an error message stating the wrong IP or path was used.

25.

Path of a network printer. There is one question that asks which of the following could be used as a path for the installation of a local printer. Which of the following is a valid path.

a. \printer\\server
b. \\server\192.168.43.27
c. \\officeserver\printername
d. ftp.printserver.com

Look for the simple path print server name followed by the printer name.
\\ always precedes the root directory. The answer is c. \\officeserver\printername

26.

Printers by URL or IP address.
A printers IP can be looked up by clicking on the information pane on the printers control panel and clicking on the information display. Printing out the network information display will include the IP address of the network printer. You would then proceed to use the Add Printer Wizard to install the network printer. All that would be needed to complete installation is to type in the correct IP address when specifying which printer.

Printers by URL are specific to http servers working on an intranet. As far as I know that A+ exam does not ask for printers by a URL extension such as http:// These questions are reserved for web servers and intranet server which are office internal http networks and these are covered in the Network+ exam.

27.

NetBEUI There is only one exam question on NetBEUI and it asks to identify what is the use of NetBEUI on a office network. These types of connections between office computers are know as protocols. Once all computers are interconnected with NetBEUI they are assigned there own NetBIOS names. The NetBIOS name identifies each individual computer on the NetBEUI network.

Question: Which of the following protocols is used on an office network to interconnect computers together over a LAN connection.

a. NetBEUI
b. NetBIOS
c. LinkSYS
d. Norton System Works

The answer is a, NetBEUI. Do not confuse with its counterpart NetBIOS. LinkSYS is the wrong answer because LinkSYS is a router, not a protocol. Norton System Works is an application not a protocol.

28.

Which of the following network protocols defines a TCP/IP network. CSMA/CD
Carrier Sense Multiple Access/ Collision Detection. This name describes packets of data moving around within a cable or broadband network in between computers. There is one other protocol that is used for wireless networks covered in the next question.

a. Carrier Sense Multiple Access/ Collision Detection
b. NetBIOS
c. File Transfer Protocol
d. IPX/ SPX

The only answer possible from the above candidates is CMSA/CD
NetBIOS identifies computers on the network.
FTP is interconnecting download from websites such as Napster. This is not a network protocol
IPX/ SPX is part of information transport and not a network protocol in itself.

Remember all we are doing on the A+ exam is defining each type of network. A+ 2007 is very much on the surface and correctly Identifying these networks will earn a nice score and a $5 per hour pay raise. Learning to configure these networks in covered on the Network+ 2007 exam.

29.

Wireless networks Avoid Collision. Carrier Sense Multiple Access/ Collision Avoidance to remember this definition, these packets are wireless and sent through the air in between wireless laptops over to wireless routers and then on to the office network. Just remember that collision is avoided as opposed to CMSA/ CD because wireless packets have plenty of room in our air current system to avoid collision.

Question: Which of the following protocols is used to connect 802.11 networks

a. CMSA/ CD
b. CMSA/ CA
c. TCP/ IP
d. WLAN

The answer is b. CMSA/ CA with the CA being for Collision Avoidance. Wireless signals have plenty of room not to collide and loose there transmission speed. CMSA/ CD is the wrong answer because CD, Collision Detection is used for overworked office networks that have trouble with being online. TCP/ IP is used for 802.3 networks. WLAN Wireless Local Area Network. WLAN consists of routers, switches, laptops trying to connect and wireless connectivity but is wrong in this case because we are only trying to define the 802.11 protocol which leaves only one answer. CMSA/ CA

30.

Which of the following network protocols is a TCP/ IP network.

a. 802.2
b. 802.3
c. 802.11

Answer: 802.3 is a TCP/ IP network. 802.11 as defined in the previous question is for wireless networks. 802.2 is an older network called Token Ring.

31.

Which of the following is a Token Ring network.

a. 802.2
b. 802.3
c. 802.11

Answer: a. 802.2 is a Token Ring network. This was a network protocol used predominately until the invention of the T1 office high speed Internet connection.

32.

Which of the following networks works at a maximum transmission speed of 11 Mbps per second

a. 802.11 a
b. 802.11 b
c. 802.11 g

Answer: b. 802.11 b works at a speed of 11 Mbps 802.11 a works at 54 Mbps 802.11g works at 54Mbps

Exam tip: This is a very difficult point about the A+ 2007 is if you are to guess a question such wrong that is not based in any reading comprehension you may automatically loose over 100 points from your total exam score. Many questions are curved because not every one learned English as there first language. A question such as this one asking to memorize pure numerical data could cost you your entire exam result.

33.

File Transfer Protocol. There are two questions on ftp on the exam. The first asks to identifying by the initials which protocol is used for transferring files in a peer to peer sharing network.

In a peer to peer network, which protocol is used to transfer files

a. ftp
b. tftp
c. sftp
d. napster

Answer: a. ftp file transfer protocol tftp is trivial file transfer protocol, which by definition is used for network with anonymous connections such as cute ftp a well known program. While fitting the definition of the question, it is marked wrong on the 2007 A+.
sftp Secure File Transfer Protocol, is ftp that requires a user name and password. This is also marked wrong on the exam. Napster, while fitting the bill for sharing files is the wrong answer because Napster was closed down by the federal authorities back in 1999 for infringing on copyright of musicians, by giving away there music as mp3's free of charge.

34.

How can I use my Internet explorer to transfer files between sites. I do not want to use a third party ftp software such as WS_FTP or Cute FTP.

Question: Which of the following commands can be used in internet explorer to transfer files?

a. ftp://username:password@domainname.com
b. ftp://domainname.com@username:password
c. http://domainname.com/username:password
d. ftp://domainname.com/username=sam:password=sloan

Answer: ftp://username:password@domainname.com ftp://at the beginning of the sentence is required, do do use any other commands such as http:// or https:// for logging into ftp servers. They will not work. Remember the username and password are separated by a colon, and the @ symbol decides where the domain name is typed in.

35.

Question: A user named Jane is using her computer without an Internet connection. She wants to browse to her My Documents folder using the Internet explorer as a file browser. Which of the following commands will browse to you 'My Documents' folder each of these answers starting with D:\ already typed into the web browser.

a. Documents and Settings\ %user account%\ My Documents
b. Documents and Settings\ %All users%\ My Documents
c. Documents and Settings\ My Documents\
d. Program Files\ Microsoft

Answer: a. The My Documents' accounts located in each individual folder archive of each user account on the computer. All of the user accounts including the All Users' account are located in the documents and settings folder. %user accounts% refers to the name of the user account, as it varies from machine to machine. Answer b. %All Users% is a wrong answer because we needed to specify Jane's user account. Answer c. is wrong because the My Documents' folder is located in the user accounts folder, not the Documents and Settings folder. Answer d. is wrong. User accounts are not located in the Program Files folder.

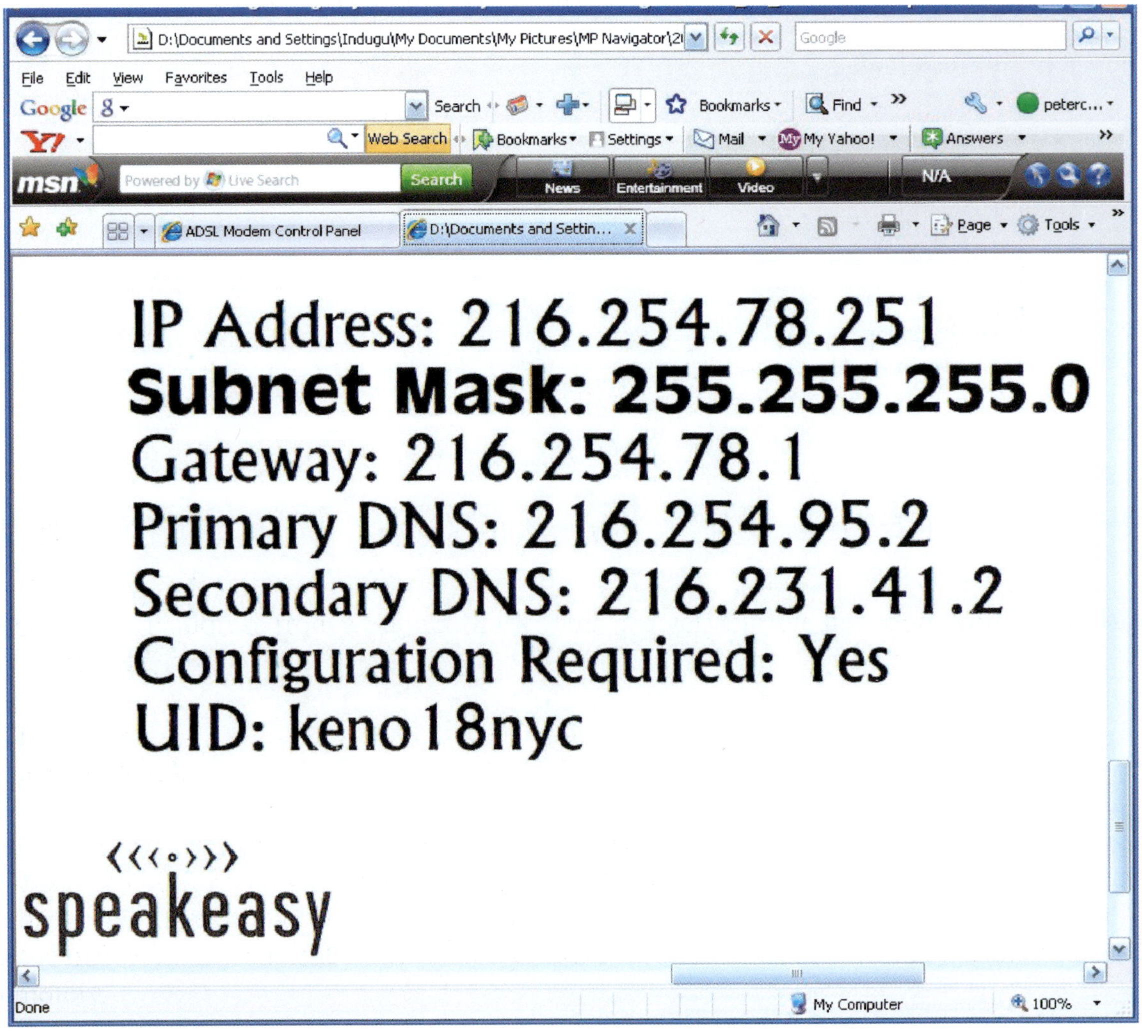

36.

Question: A user from your office accounting department complains that when he uses his Internet explorer his computer terminates abruptly. His applications all freeze and loose there data. You need to uninstall and reinstall your Internet explorer without using the Windows XP Professional CD.

Answer: Click Start< Control Panel< Add or Remove Programs< Click Add or Remove windows components< allow windows components wizard to run< uncheck the Internet explorer icon< Click next< Click OK

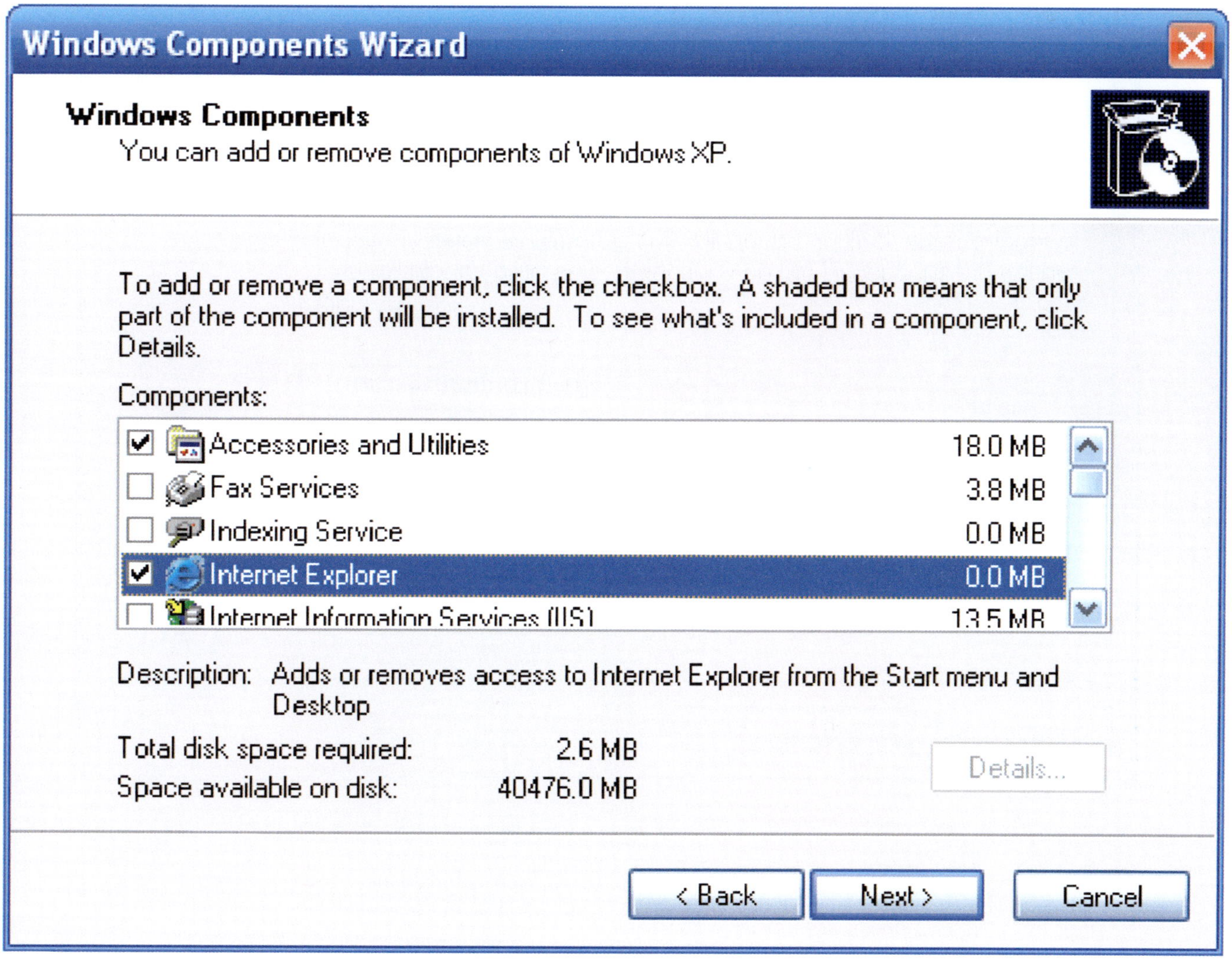

37.

Question: You are using a recently installed copy of Windows XP Professional, and you keep getting an error message that you firewall is turned off. What is the path to use to turn on windows firewall using the Control Panel?

Answer: Click Start< Control Panel< Windows Firewall< Select the green On radio tab< Check the box< Don't allow exceptions< Click OK

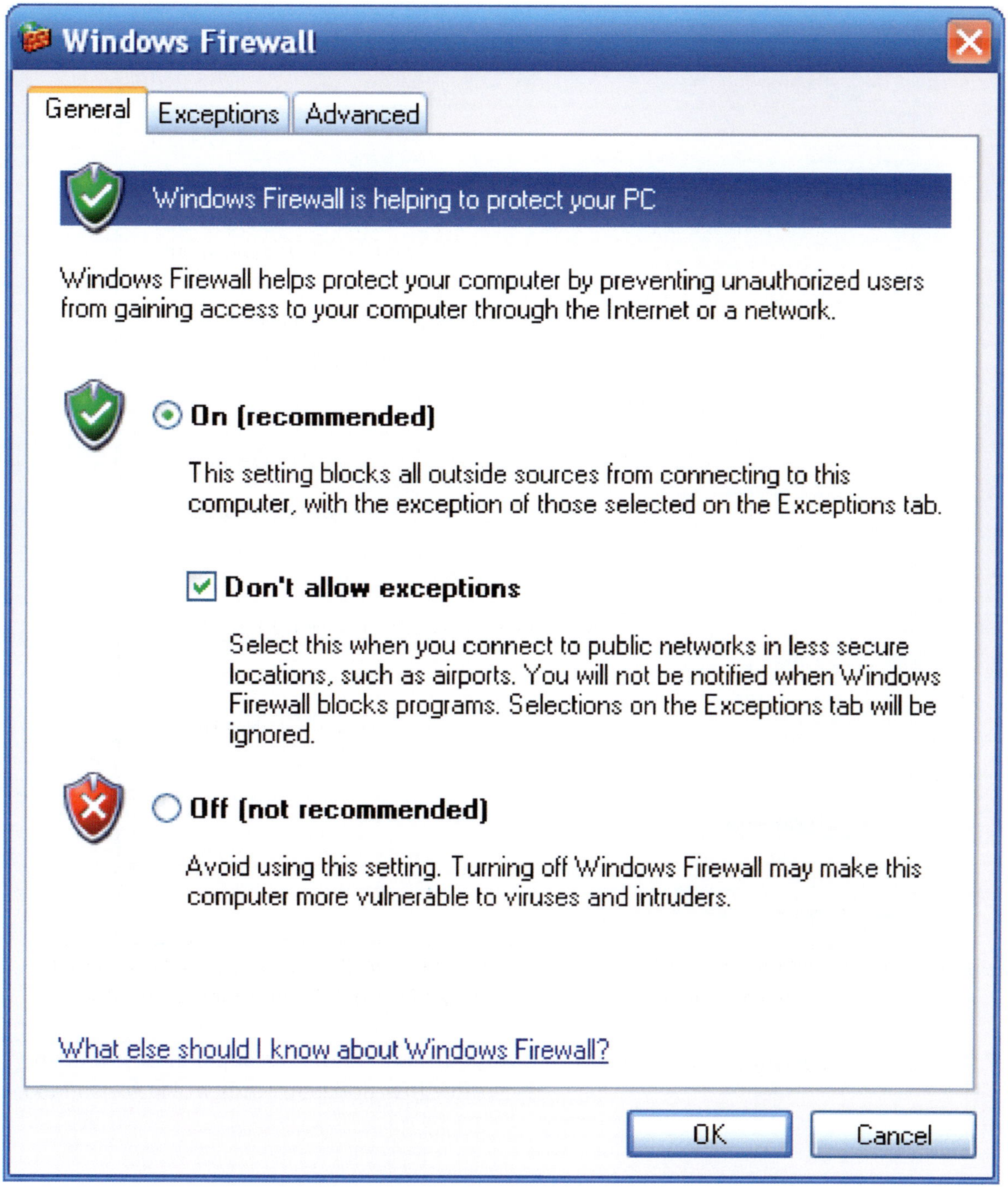

38.

Question: You have installed Norton Anti Virus and have detected a firewall conflict with the Generic Windows Firewall. Using the Taskbar (not the control panel) open the windows security center and disable the firewall.

Answer: Click the taskbar Windows Security Icon

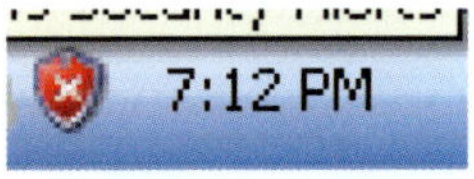

Double click on the red X shaped like a shield, the following screen will open.

Click the Windows Firewall hyperlink<

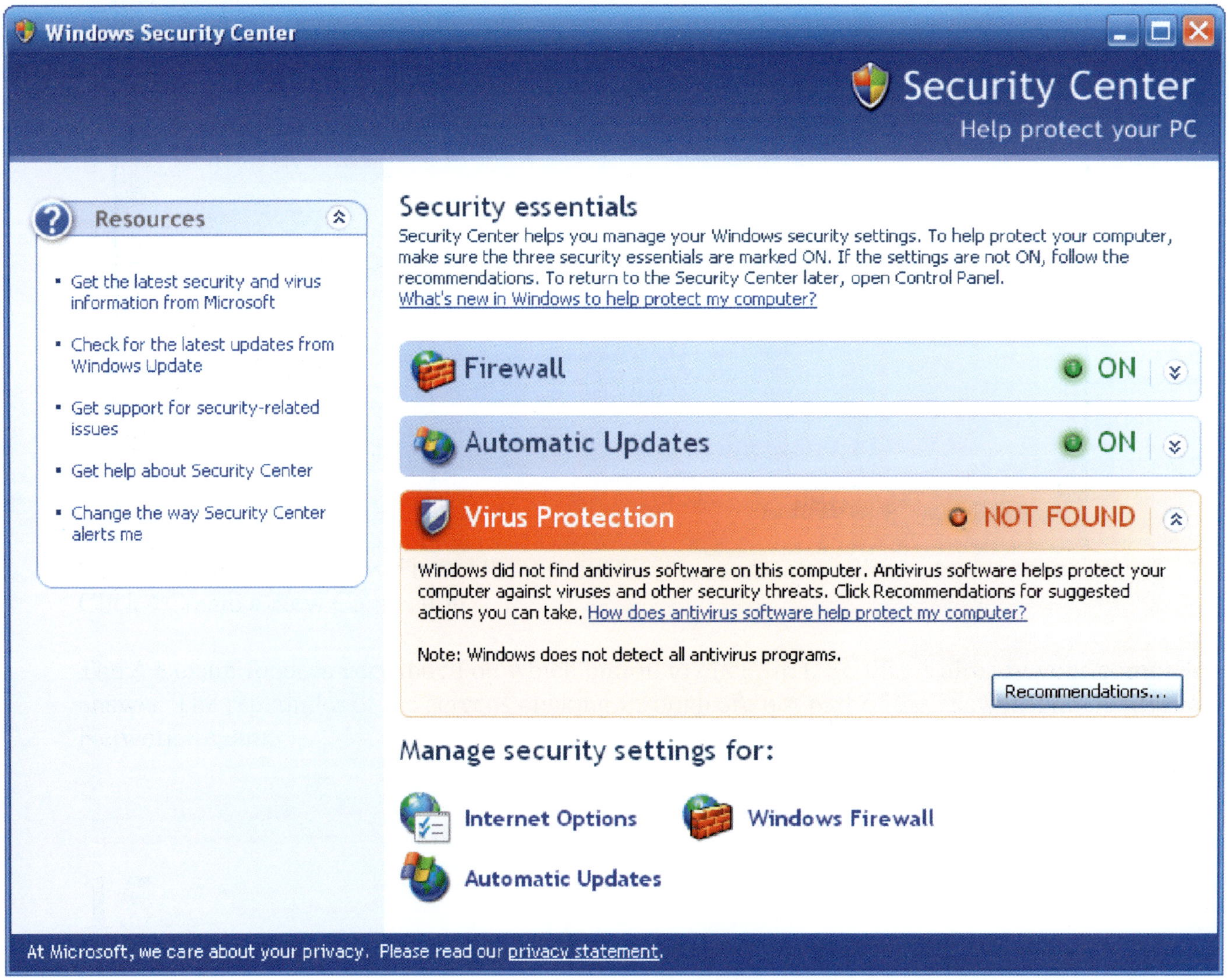

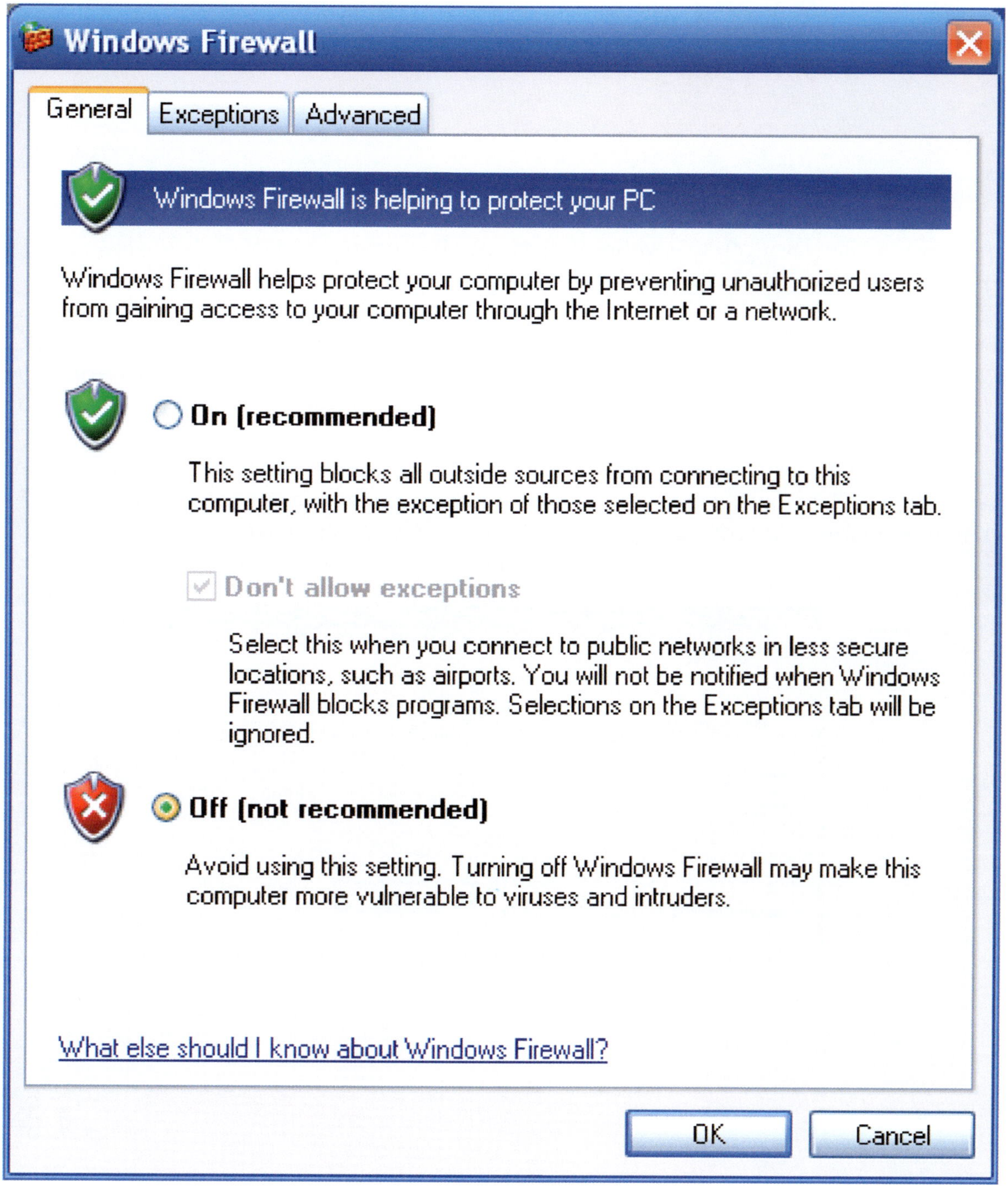

Select the Off radio button< Click OK< restart your computer and your Norton ant virus will take over.

39.

Question: You need to install using your windows CD What is the correct path to take?

Answer: Insert the Windows XP Professional CD< Wait for the CD to run automatically< Click Install optional Windows components< wait for the Windows components wizard to load

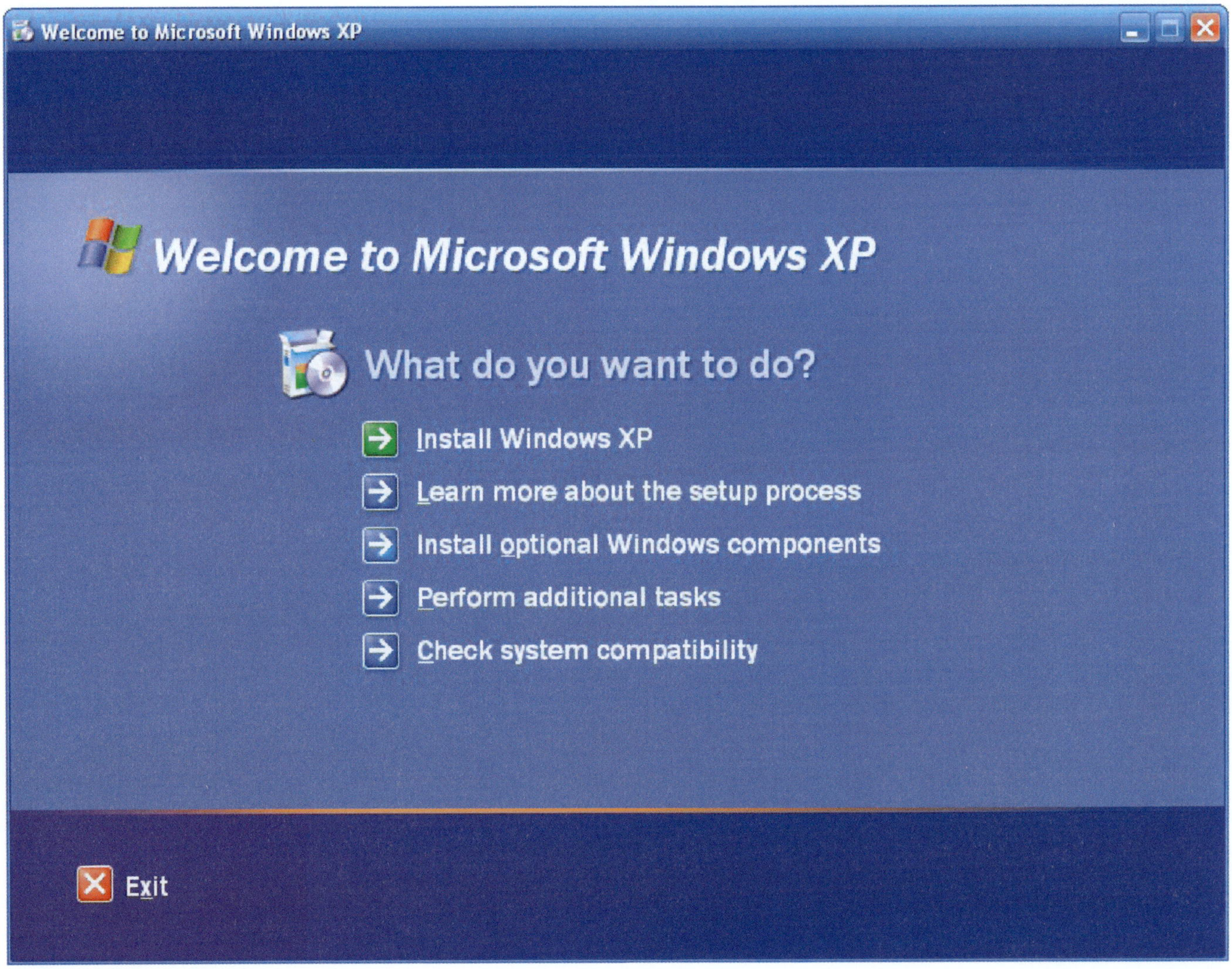

40.

Question: How do I open the command prompt in Windows XP Professional

a. Start< Run< type CMD< press enter
b. Start< Run< type MSConfig.exe< press enter
c. Start< Run< type Ipconfig /all< press enter
d. Start< Run< type CMD< press enter< type ping< press enter

Answer: a. The command prompt is open by typing CMD into the command prompt. Another way to open the command prompt is by typing Command.exe . CMD is an abbreviation of command. Ipconfig /all is used to look up the entire IP configuration of a computer and only after the command prompt is open.

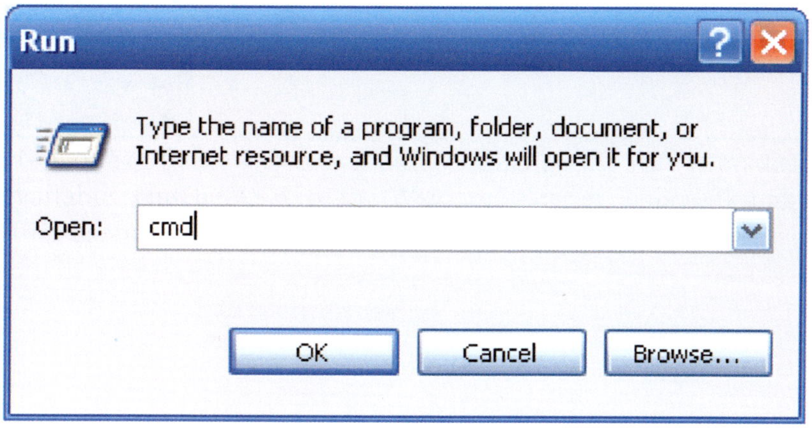

41.

Question: How do I edit the boot.ini file in Windows XP Professional

a. Start< Run< MSConfig.exe< press enter
b. Start< Run< CMD< press enter
c. Start< Run< Sysprep.exe< press enter
d. Start< Run< Autoexec.bat< press enter

Answer: a. MSConfig.exe when typed into the command prompt will open in its own window. From this panel you can edit the boot.ini have your computer start in safe mode with /SAFEBOOT, use the /BASEVIDEO to load windows without the video drivers for troubleshooting you VGA driver. If you need to load you computer without SCSI support for a

hard drive use /SOS, if you need a log of all programs and there operations upon startup use /BOOTLOG, to load windows without using the graphical user interface use /NOGUIBOOT file control which programs are run at startup, which programs.
Sysprep.exe is located in the I386 folder on your Windows XP CD not in the root directory of your C: drive so your cannot run from using the c: CMD prompt . Autoexec.bat is not an executable file so it cannot be loaded at all from the command prompt. Be aware this is a trick answer and appears several times on the A+ 2007 exam as an incorrect answer.

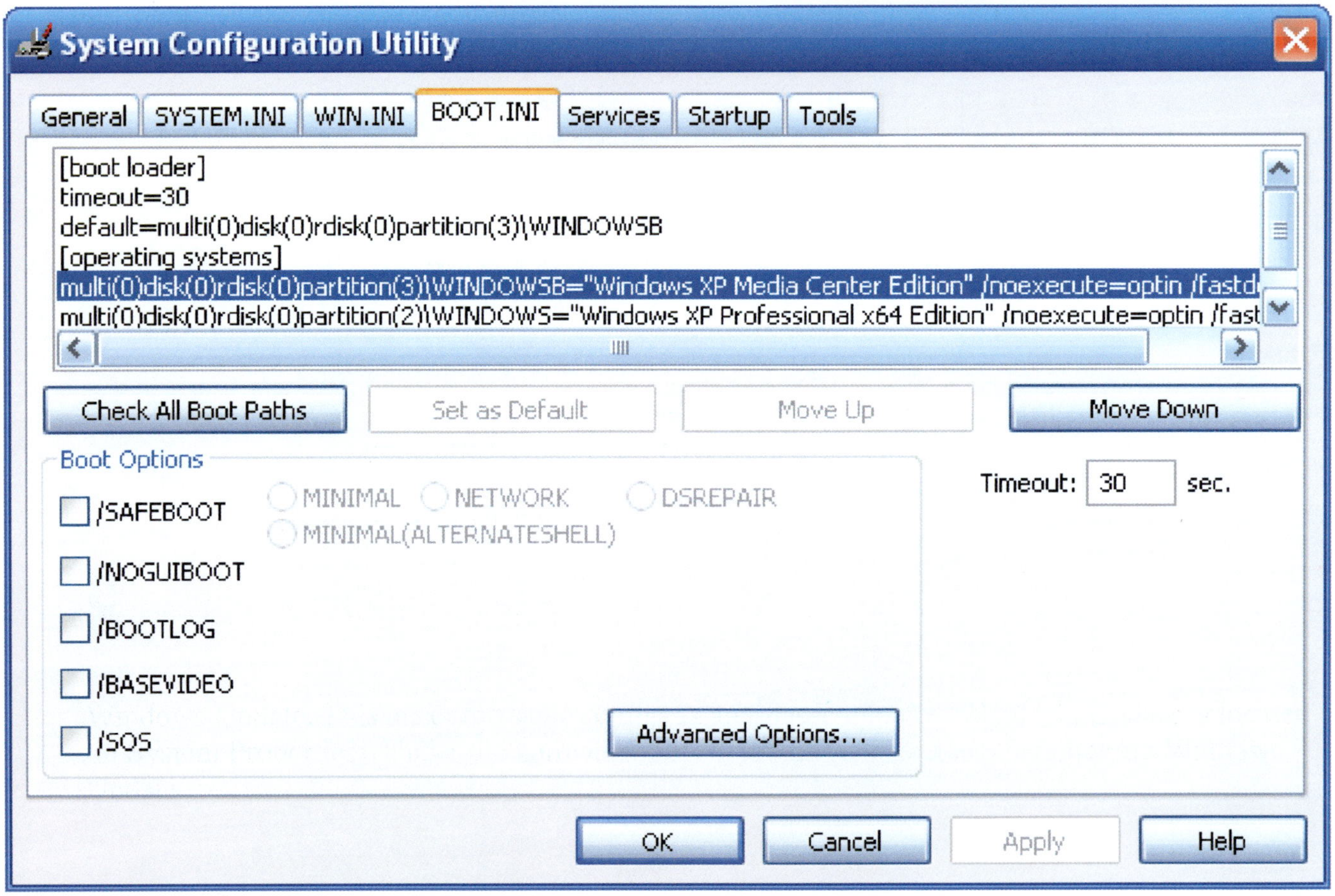

42.

Question: A user in your office is using her computer when the display starts flickering. She cannot comfortably read the screen of her word processing application. You tried to roll back the driver using the Device Manager but the problem persists. What command can you use to start the the computer using the generic video driver and then install a new driver from that point on.

Answer: Click< Start< Run< Msconfig< press enter< click the Boot.ini tab< check the box /BASEVIDEO< click apply< when the prompt appears click yes< Click OK< restart the computer.

43.

You are a Field Technician on a routine call to inspect a computer for difficulty. You notice that when the computer starts up there are many unnecessary programs running. You restart the computer one time and the machine takes an abnormally long time to load the basic startup programs. The user asks you to stop all of these programs from launching on startup except for Norton and Instant Messenger. You need to remedy the problem without uninstalling these programs. What do you do?

Answer: Click< Start< Run< Msconfig< press enter< Click the Startup tab< uncheck the programs you do not want to run at startup< Click apply< Click OK at the prompt< Click OK< Restart the computer.

44.

Question: You have installed Norton Anti Virus but there is a conflict with another Anti Virus software named AVG. You need to install AVG anti virus before Norton can run properly. What is the path used to uninstall a software?

Answer: Click Start< Control Panel< Add or Remove Programs< select AVG from the list< Click Change Remove

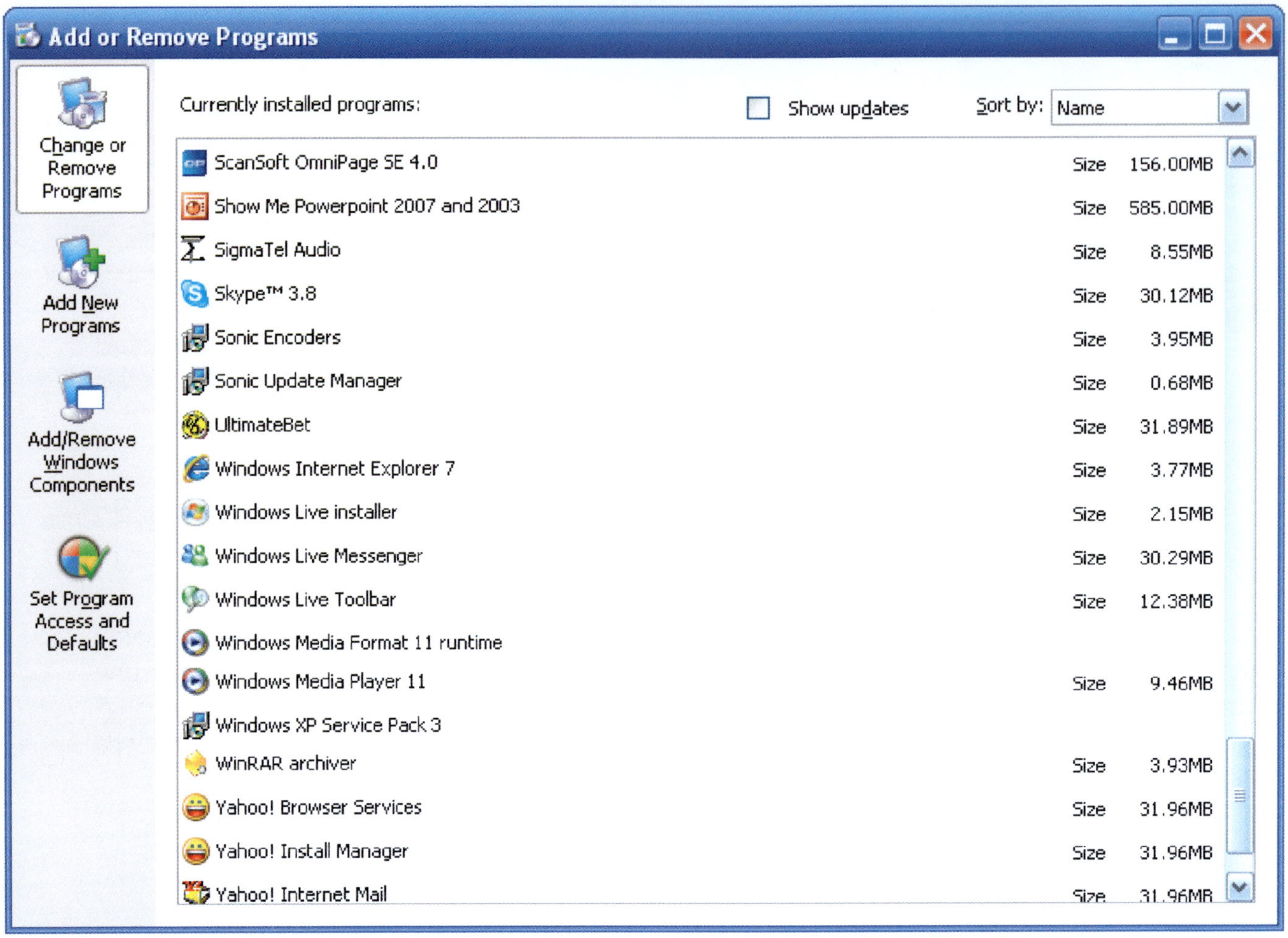

45.

Question: how do I run a program in Windows XP Professional.

Answer: Click< Start< Run

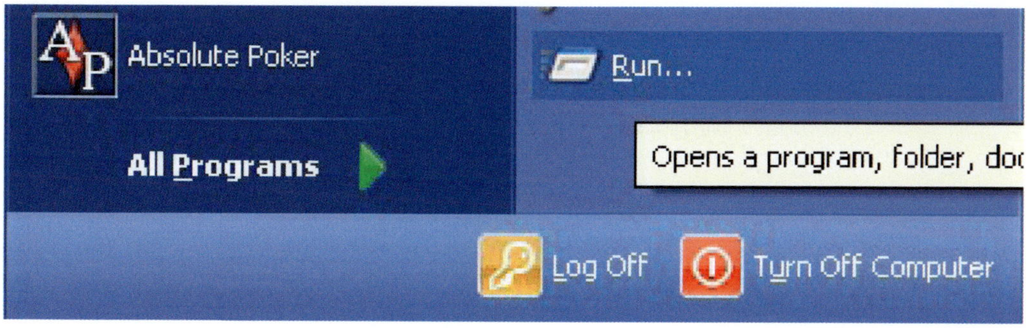

That is an actual question on the exam, so As easy as it sounds to click Start< Run, you have to remember the path that was used, clicking the sequence of both buttons, and the it did not involve double clicking on any application.

46.

Question: Which of the following programs causes a compact disk to run automatically at startup?

a. Autorun.exe
b. Setup.exe
c. Autorun.swf
d. Autorun.fla

Answer: a. Autorun.exe will cause the cd to launch its presentation as soon as being entered into the cd rom drive. Many cd's have autorun.exe files these days, you can even make your own powerpoint presentations to load automatically with autorun.exe on a windows computer. Answer b. Setup.exe is incorrect and this would install a program but only after being clicked on. We are looking for a program that runs automatically. Answer c. Autorun.swf is wrong also. swf is the extension of a flash file. Swf is an animation file for the web that can be used on cd's as well, but does not have the same function as autorun. Answer: d. is also wrong. .fla files are work files associated with Macromedia Flash software. These files are saved to be able to edit artwork and animation documents by the artist and designers.

47.

Which of the following file extensions is an executable file?

a. exe
b. inf
c. ini
d. bat

Answer: a. exe stands for executable file. Answer b. is wrong inf is an information file of system information. Answer c. ini is wrong. Ini is a configuration file that keeps information such which drivers are used to load which software. Answer d. is wrong bat are batch files. Batch files contain information specific to how programs load and what memory is allocated. Batch files are covered in depth when studying for microsoft certification.

48.

Question: A CPA in the accounting department wants to log onto her assistants user account without closing down her programs or applications. Momentarily check on an excel spreadsheet typed up by her assistant and then go back to using her regular user account. What path should she use?

Answer: Click< Start< Log Off< Switch User

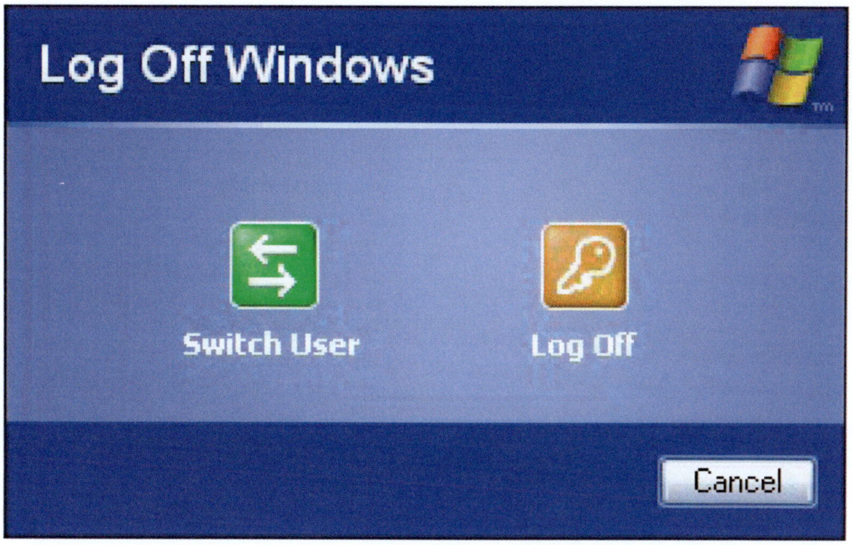

49.

Question: Using the command prompt what is the command you can use to view the entire ip configuration of a computer running Windows XP Professional.

Answer: Click Start< Run< CMD< press enter< type Ipconfig /all< press enter

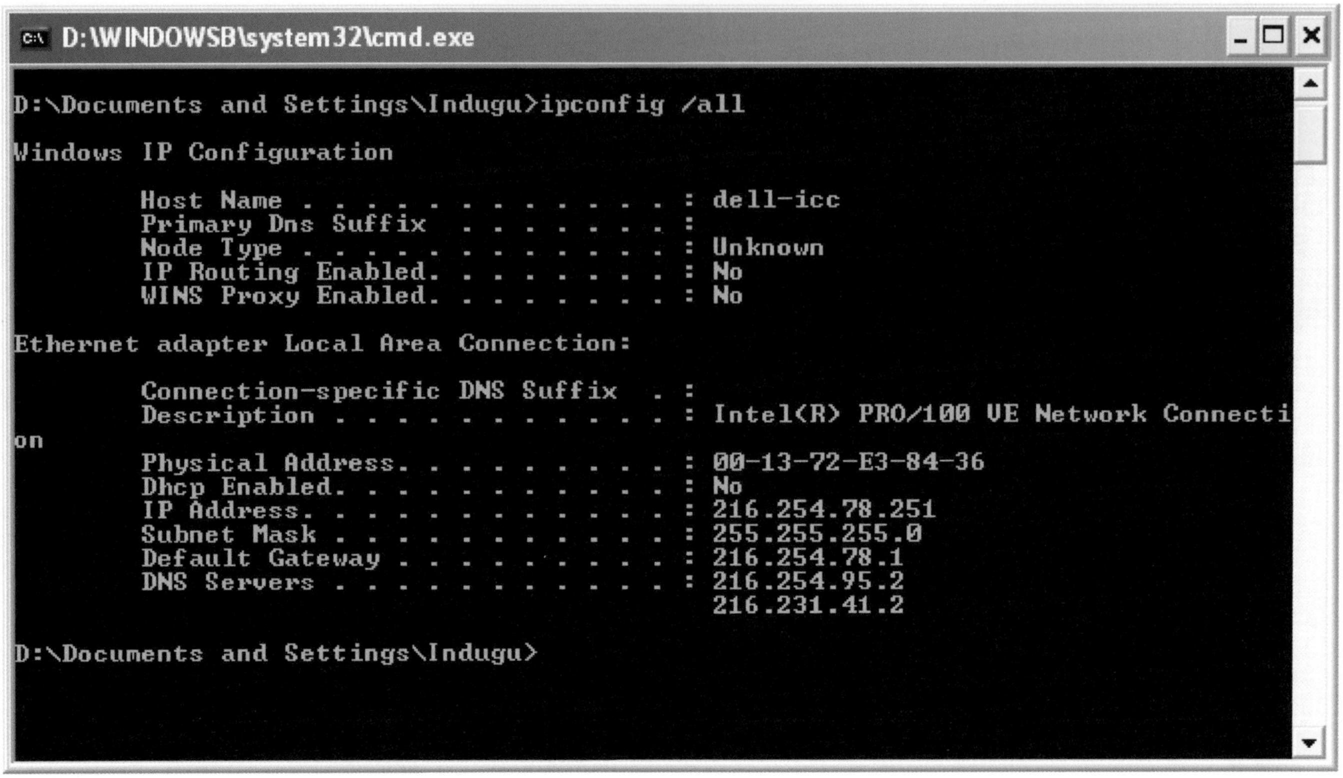

50.

Question: What command can be used at the command prompt to test the connection to a specific IP address?

Answer: Click< Start< Run< type CMD< type ping %ip address%
This will display a page of information about that connectivity to the IP address you have sent the ping echo request. Ping is most commonly used to test out connections around an office building. Two computers connected on a subnet through a common switch can ping one another to test connectivity. Someone in an office would commonly ping an office printer to make sure the connection is working correctly. The third use of ping is to check connection to website that would otherwise not be loading, for example
ping yahoo.com would check the connection from your computer to the yahoo.com website. Ping is the most basic ms-dos command but has many uses keeping a computers connection regularly checked.

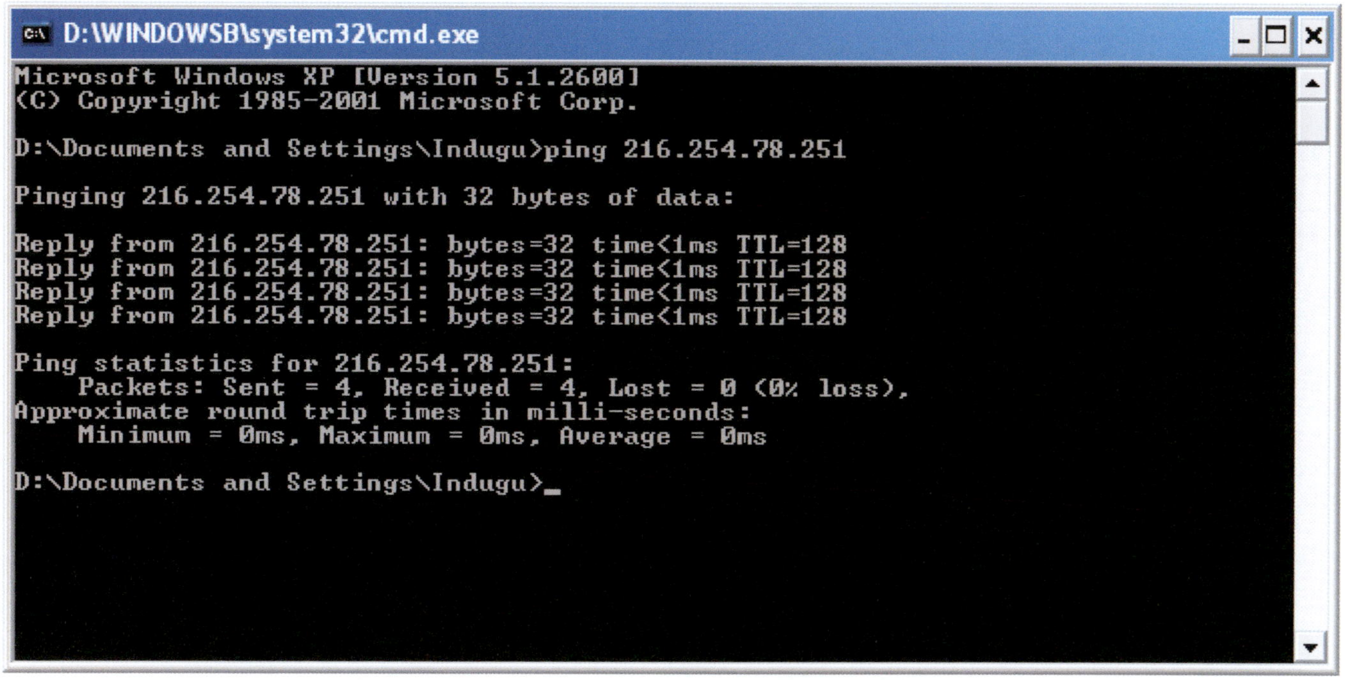

Thank you very much for reading my first IT computer book. Best luck on your A+ 2007 exam

Sam Sloan

Printed in Dunstable, United Kingdom

91220869R00025